UNBREATHABLE BREATHE

(a cystic fibrosis patients)

Morgan A. Grass

Description

- Introduces readers to the symptoms, causes, day-to-day activities of people with cystic fibrosis (CF), how the disease affects the body, and what it's like to live with the condition.
- Things that provide joy and affection to CFers
- What to do as a CFer to keep healthy.

It's critical to gain as much knowledge as you can about cystic fibrosis and how to handle it if you have it. Serious infections may be avoided by making an effort to maintain your health as much as possible and by seeking treatment when necessary. The disease cystic fibrosis is incurable. Even while it may not be feasible to completely eliminate flare-ups, there are steps you can do to lessen their frequency and intensity as well as enhance your quality of life.

Keywords

- Cystic fibrosis
- Adventurer & Explorer Biographies
- True Crime
- Genetic Disorders & Diseases
- The crushing desire to freeze time and isolate yourself
- The unstable phase of "firsts" — first holidays, birthdays, adventure
- Feeling left out
- CF Permission to grief

Category

- Cystic Fibrosis
- Immune Systems
- Attention for cystic Fibrosis patient

Table of contents

As a cystic fibrosis sufferer, a sixteen-year-old girl spends the majority of her time in the hospital. She still tries to live like every other normal child, but she lives in anguish and fear knowing that her life is worth not living again. She developed the illness when she was a little child and has since lived each day as if there would be no tomorrow. She has strict rules, boundaries, and self-control in her life.

CHAPTER ONE

Cystic Fibrosis: What Is It?

Being a hereditary illness, cystic fibrosis (CF) is something you inherit from your parents at birth. It has an impact on how your body produces mucus, a fluid that supports the operation of your organs and systems. When you have CF, your mucus becomes thick and glue-like instead of being thin and slick like it should be. This obstructs ducts and tubes all over your body.

This heavy mucus accumulates inside your airways over time. Breathing is challenging as a result. Infections are caused by the mucus, which collects microorganisms. Additionally, it can result in serious lung damage such as fibrosis and cysts (fluid-filled sacs) (scar tissue). CF gained its name in this manner.

Cystic fibrosis affects more than 30,000 people in the United States. Each year, doctors identify roughly 1,000 new instances

Symptoms of Cystic Fibrosis

CF patients may have symptoms like:

- Constipation issues or frequently occurring, oily stools
- respiratory issues such as wheezing
- lung infections that are common
- male infertility in particular
- Problems gaining weight or growing
- Skin with a strong salty flavor

Causes of Cystic Fibrosis

Cystic fibrosis is brought on by a mutation in the CFTR gene (cystic fibrosis transmembrane conductance regulator). This gene regulates the movement of fluids and salt into and out of your cells. When the CFTR gene isn't functioning properly, your body produces a buildup of sticky mucus.

You must inherit the gene with the mutation from both of your parents in order to develop CF. Ninety percent of persons who are affected have the F508del mutation in at least one copy.

If you have just one copy, you won't show any signs of the illness, but you will be a carrier anyway. Therefore, there is a possibility that you will pass it on to your offspring.

Approximately 10 million Americans have CF. Every time two CF carriers have a baby, there's a 25% (1 in 4) chance that their baby will be born with CF.

The following organs are also affected by cystic fibrosis:

1. Pancreas: Your pancreas' ducts are blocked by the thick mucus brought on by CF. This prevents digestive enzymes, which are proteins that help

break down food, from getting to your intestine. Your body thus struggles to obtain the nutrition it requires. Diabetes may develop as a result of this over time.

2. Liver: Your liver becomes inflamed if the channels used to drain bile get blocked. This may result in cirrhosis, a severe scarring condition.

3. Small intestine: The lining of the small intestine can deteriorate because high-acid foods from your stomach can be challenging to digest.

4. Large intestine: Your stomach's heavy fluid may cause your excrement to be bulky and challenging to pass. Blockages may result from this. In some cases, your intestine may also start to fold in on itself like an accordion,a condition called intussusception.

5. Bladder: Chronic or long-lasting coughing weakens your bladder

muscles. Almost 65% of women with CF have stress incontinence.

On a wonderful morning, I woke up struggling to breathe. It was more like the air in my room had frozen over, making it impossible for me to scream. As my mother entered the room to perform her regular duties, she noticed that I was barely breathing. Because it seemed so foreign to her, she was unable to panic. I was unable to respond because I wasn't present when she asked, "Nora, what's wrong with you?" She hurried me to the hospital, and after various tests, the doctor informed my mother that I have a fatal illness (cystic fibrosis).My mom and my siblings wept for me because my dad wasn't with us anymore; they all knew I would pass very shortly. There are restrictions on what I can accomplish on a daily basis due to my health and medications that impact me (the majority of persons with CF wouldn't live to reach their 18th birthday). For instance, I don't always have the same amount of energy; some days I can get through the day easily, and other days I tire quickly. Although it is irritating, I am making an effort to cope and accept it.

I just have to make do with what I have because it's not my fault that my body is built this way.

I can still do a lot despite having CF, like play the guitar and sing

Everyday living with CF

My morning routine includes an hour or more of self-care, which begins with using an inhaler to widen my airways. The mucus that had accumulated in my lungs over night was then released and cleared using a treatment vest (it could be vibrating and really relieving).

In order to minimize edema and loosen the sticky mucus in my lungs and make it simpler for me to cough up and clear my airways, I then combine nebulizer treatments with drugs. Antibiotics may occasionally be used in conjunction with these therapies to treat inflammatory infections. The objective is to improve breathing and increase airflow to my lungs.

After that, it's time to eat, take a shower, and go to class. My schedule is full of lectures and rehearsal and singing

CHAPTER TWO

My visits

I receive evaluations and care from a variety of professionals at the Cystic Fibrosis Center at each of my visits, including:

- Attending doctors

During CF office hours, the staff attending physician discusses my condition with members of the healthcare team and establishes goals for my treatment moving forward with my mother and the team.

The attending physician for the inpatient service will choose my medical care throughout any hospital stays. Every month, the attending switches roles. The entire pulmonary team meets regularly to discuss and organize the inpatient care. Advanced practice nurses

During CF office hours, the nurse practitioner reviews my status with members of the healthcare team and together with my mom and the team develops goals for future care. When CFers at home have medical or nursing questions, the calls will frequently be answered by nurse practitioners between 9 a.m. and 4:30 p.m. Nurse practitioners along with the attending physician are also responsible for coordinating the inpatient care during hospitalization.

- Pulmonary associate

During the three years of the fellowship training, the pulmonary fellow is tasked with providing primary CF care for patients alongside the attending physician during CF office hours. In addition, the fellows alternate every month on the inpatient ward to provide care for children who are admitted for overnight stays and weekend visits.

The on-call outpatient fellow works alongside the attending physician to provide outpatient emergency treatment on evenings, weekends, and holidays. During this time, the person answers phones and gives

instructions to the emergency room staff should your child be seen there.
pediatrician in training
According to the Pulmonary Team's instructions, the pediatric resident provides inpatient patients with daily medical care.

- Admin nurse

The outpatient visit's treatment is coordinated by the office nurse, a registered or licensed practical nurse. The office nurse's duties may include gathering and recording patients' height and weight, giving injections, instructing patients on how to use inhalers properly, and setting up special tests during clinics.

- Principal nurse

The registered nurse in charge of organizing and planning your child's care during their hospital stay is known as the primary nurse. On the inpatient facilities, a group of nurses collaborate closely with the primary nurse to care for your kid.

- Physical therapist

The role of the physical therapist (PT) in Cystic Fibrosis Center includes teaching chest physical therapy (CPT) and alternative breathing techniques to children and their families. These techniques are reviewed annually. Also, the PT assists in obtaining equipment related to CPT (e.g., wedges, mechanical percussors, vest).

During hospitalizations the PT evaluates exercise tolerance and develops a program suitable to the child's physical and medical needs as well as interest. Generally, a child will be seen three times a week for exercise including general stretching and warm-up, aerobic activity (chosen by the child) and cool down/breathing exercises.

During hospital stays, the PT assesses exercise tolerance and creates a program tailored to the child's interests, physical needs, and medical requirements. A kid will typically be seen three times per week for physical therapy, which includes general stretches and warm-ups, an aerobic activity of the child's choosing, and cool-down/breathing exercises.

- The social worker

The social worker holds a Master's degree in Social Work from graduate school (MSW). A social worker with expertise and awareness of the effects of chronic illness on people, families, and other systems, such as schools and peer groups. She can help with emotional support and stress management related to a chronic condition. The social worker also has knowledge of community and medical facilities that can offer functioning family support services

- Nutritionist

The nutritionist's job is to teach parents techniques that will help the child grow as optimally as possible through healthy eating. This is done by regularly measuring things like height, weight, and food intake as well as evaluating things like enzyme replacement treatment and other dietary supplements.

To assist children with CF consume a diet that is suitable for their age and physical needs, information about optimal nutrition is offered, along with suggestions for how it might be improved. Treatment recommendations take into account the child's food choices, family eating habits, cultural background, and socioeconomic position.

CHAPTER THREE

What it's like to live with CF; How CF affects daily life

We constantly encounter unpleasant situations, frustrating encounters, guilt, mistaken obligation, and misconceptions. I believe most people with cystic fibrosis have at some point or another thought, "I wish people knew _____ about my life with CF." Simply put, unless you actually live with CF, it's nearly impossible for people to grasp what our lives are really like.

Even our closest friends and family don't entirely comprehend because they are unable to share our emotions.

Due to the wide range of CF from person to person, there are even significant knowledge gaps between two people who have the same CF.But being aware of some crucial facts can aid in closing the gap.

Here are a few details regarding my life with CF that I wish people were aware of.

I wish people would realize that CF affects a person on more than just a physical level. CF also affects one's mental and emotional well-being. Living with cystic fibrosis involves several challenges, including managing the physical restrictions caused by the condition, adjusting to a decreased life expectancy, and occasionally dealing with a lower quality of life. Understanding this is crucial, but sadly, treating mental health conditions is only just starting to take center stage in CF care.

I wish people thought they could question me. I think Claire Wineland gave others the courage to open many doors that they were afraid to knock on because she was so honest about her life and her illness. Since my second-grade diagnosis, I have never wanted anyone to feel like they couldn't ask me questions about cystic fibrosis (CF) because it is the only way to dispel myths. I always appreciate sincere curiosity or interest. I'm not embarrassed to have CF, and your willingness to bring up the matter demonstrates to me your concern for me. But if you ask, do pay attention.

I wish friends were aware of how quickly I get sick. Please, please, please don't come near me if you are even a little ill, especially in the cold. People with CF are extremely prone to illness. To you, it might only seem like a small cough and runny nose, but if I get what you have, I can be sick for weeks as I fight to recover from that "little" cold. If you cancel arrangements because you're feeling under the weather, I won't get upset. This danger is increased for those whose CF is more severe than mine or for those who have had a lung transplant. A little virus or cold may necessitate hospitalization and perhaps result in demise.

I wish my friends understood why I don't make plans with them. In college, I was usually able to keep up with my friends when we went out drinking (I don't advise it, though). If I'm being honest, I really do enjoy a glass of wine or cups of yogurt; but now, having more than one drink makes me feel like absolute crap. Therefore, I usually avoid social scenes because the pressure to keep up by drinking copious amounts and staying up past my 10 p.m. bedtime just isn't worth my lungs getting sick and my body feeling tired and achy for days. Instead of sleeping all day, I would much rather get up at a decent time on a Saturday, go for a run, and spend the day hanging out with my mom or siblings. If you want to make time for our friendship, let's do something that isn't focused around drinking all night -- really, let's do anything else!

I wish people understood why I make certain decisions. CF has a way of helping you prioritize your life; I'm always thinking about what is most important to me. At the top of my list are spending time with my family, taking care of my health, seeing the world, and making a positive impact on the people in my life and our planet. I have a pretty low threshold for things that don't matter to me or things that feel like a waste of time.

CHAPTER FOUR

It can be hard to know exactly what to do to support patients with CF when you aren't sure what they are going through.
My family is really trying their best to make me feel loved and never left out. I just want to make a list of what we CF patients really love because I know that we all (CF patients) feel the same way.

1. Bring, prepare, or buy us a meal.
Most people with CF need to consume a ridiculous amount of calories to fight infection and sustain our bodies, which work extra hard to function. Frustratingly, cooking can require a lot of physical and mental energy that on some days we just don't have readily available, especially when sick. I always feel so loved when my mom or friends provide a meal for me.

2. Clean our nebulizer cups.
Growing up, my mom boils my nebulizer cups to clean them. She even cleaned them

when I came home from college on breaks or returns from the hospital.Help a CFer out, and they will thank you!

3. Offer to help check off an item on our to-do list.
I don't know about others with CF, but I feel like my to-do list is constantly growing. Between refilling medications, fighting insurance battles, scheduling doctor's appointments, and all the other "normal people" stuff, I never get to the bottom of that dang thing. But my siblings are really the best

4. Offer to help carry groceries, heavy items, etc.
People with CF can't breathe very well. Guess what? Carrying heavy items just makes us more breathless. Offering to carry groceries, heavy boxes, etc. when you can help us save the extra energy needed to complete other necessary activities of daily living.

5. Continue to invite us to places even if we have declined or canceled in the past.

FOMO (fear of missing out) is a real disorder, and I suffer from it 100 percent. CF gets in the way of my social life a lot of the time. Whether it's IVs, fatigue, or hospital stays, facets of CF prevent me from spending time with the people I love. I always feel truly cared for when I am invited out (again) after declining or canceling previously.

6. Don't ask us, 'How are you doing?' Ask, 'How can I help you?' and 'What are you struggling with?'

When someone asks me, "How are you doing?" I struggle to answer and usually settle on something like,"I'm doing well. Hanging in there. I wasn't feeling too well last week, but I feel much better this week." I don't want to blatantly lie, but I also don't want to be a Negative Nancy in my response. If you really want to know how we are doing, use more intentional and direct questions that give us an opportunity to talk about our current experiences without relying on a cliché response.

7. Ignore our cough.
Ugh, the cough. I know I am with true understanding spirits when I erupt into a coughing fit and no one stops the conversation or pays any attention to the red face and horrible coughing expression. Please, just ignore the coughing (unless we are on the floor or puking) and give us time to calm down and resume as normal. We are totally fine!

8. Encourage us to stay compliant with medication (and congratulate us when we are).
CFers get a bad rap for being medically noncompliant, meaning we don't do what we are supposed to do. I have issues with this reputation because the general population can't even drink the recommended amount of water on any given day, but people with CF are expected to take 50 pills a day,

complete hours of breathing treatments, consume thousands of calories, monitor blood sugar, and never miss a beat. It is difficult to be medically compliant. Every. Single. Day. We need encouragement, and we need someone to acknowledge the work we put into staying healthy.

9. Gift ideas: gift cards to restaurants, gummy bears, words of support, and understanding.
If you need to get us a gift, gift cards to food establishments are always appreciated. Patients can use them while in the hospital or when we are too sick to cook. Also, I don't know why this is, but CFers love gummy bears. There must be some sort of gummy bear mutation. Give us a 5-pound bag of Haribo Gold-Bears, and we feel all kinds of feelings. Lastly, some days I simply need a friend to tell me they might not fully understand what I am experiencing, but they support me. Words of encouragement, admiration, and respect can promote healing

and drive when in the thick of a brutal disease.

And this is especially to all CFers like me. Please let your mind guide you. All you ever need in this life is already in you. We only need to learn to trust in life and how to open our hearts to the new and unknown. To listen carefully to our inner voice and let it guide us.

To all CFers

Today, people with cystic fibrosis (CF) live longer, healthier lives than ever before. If you have CF, medications and treatments can help you manage your disease. You can also take many actions -- big and small – that will make a difference in how you feel. Here are five things you can do to live your healthiest, fullest life.

1. Avoid Germs

You need to be on germ patrol at all times. CF causes thick, sticky mucus to build up in your lungs, creating an environment where germs thrive. This can put you at risk for lung infections, which affect how well your lungs work. They can also cause lung disease to get worse.

Follow these tips to steer clear of germs in your day-to-day life:

- Stay at least 6 feet away from anyone who's sick.

- Avoid activities that put you near other people with CF, to lower the risk of spreading sickness.
- Frequently wash your hands with soap and water.
-
- Clean and disinfect your medical equipment properly.
- Don't share items that come into contact with saliva (straws or utensils) with other people -- even family.
- Avoid contact with dust or dirt.
- Stay current on your vaccines, including the flu vaccine, and ask family and friends to do the same.

2. Exercise

Between feeling tired, out of breath, and coughing, you may wonder whether exercise is a good idea when you have CF. Not only is it OK to exercise, but doctors recommend it. Exercise helps clear mucus out of your lungs. It strengthens your heart and muscles. The stronger you feel, the easier it is to do everyday tasks. Choose activities that you enjoy and that keep you moving.

Work with your CF care team to find an exercise program that works best for you. Try to do moderate exercise for about 20 minutes every day of the week. This means you can still talk while you move. Add resistance training, like lifting weights, 1 or 2 days per week.

If you go to the gym, take steps to avoid germs. For instance:

- Wipe down equipment with an alcohol-based gel before you use it.
- Wash your hands after you touch any surface -- from treadmills to hairdryers.
- Stay at least 6 feet away from anyone who's sick.

3. Eat Well

With CF, the pancreas doesn't work as it should. It doesn't make the enzymes it needs to help digest food. This affects how well your body gets nutrients. You use more energy to breathe, fight infections, and maintain your weight than other people do. That's why people who have CF often need about twice the calories the average person needs in a day. Work with your CF care team to find out how many daily calories you need and the best way to get them.

4. Take Care of Your Emotional Health

When you have CF, your physical health takes center stage. But your emotional health is important, too. Because you have a chronic (ongoing) disease, you may face lots of stress and anxiety. This can put you at risk for depression. When you feel anxious or depressed, you may not take care of yourself as well as you should. If you have any signs of anxiety or depression, seek help. Some of the signs include:

- Sadness
- Low energy
- Feeling hopeless or worthless
- Difficulty concentrating
- Frequent crying
- Irritability

Depression can also cause problems with your sleep. You may sleep too much or too little. Or you might worry a lot and have headaches. You may even have thoughts of suicide.

If you think you may be anxious or depressed, talk to someone on your CF care team. Working with a mental health professional, like a psychologist, can make a big difference in how you feel.

5. Learn About Your Fertility and Sexual Health

Men with CF are missing the vas deferens. This is a part of the male reproductive system. Sperm travel through it to exit the penis during ejaculation. Most men with CF make healthy sperm, but they're infertile (can't get a woman pregnant).

If you're a man with CF, you and your partner can conceive with the help of assisted reproductive technology. Ask your doctor for a referral to a urologist -- a doctor who specializes in male reproductive organs. They can find out whether you're infertile and help you take the next steps toward having a baby.

Most women with CF are fertile, but the disease can make it harder to get pregnant. They have thicker cervical mucus, which is harder for sperm to travel through to reach the egg. But most women with CF who want to get pregnant are able to and can go on to have a normal pregnancy.

You can also have a normal, healthy sex life when you have CF. Keep in mind that you can still be at risk for unplanned pregnancies and sexually transmitted diseases (STDs). If you're not ready to have children or you're with a partner who hasn't been tested for STDs, always use birth control, such as condoms.